BALANCE EXERCISES FOR SENIORS

Low-impact exercise for senior mobility and fitness

Lucas Olle

kindly notice the material provided inside this booklet is for educational use only. utmost attempt has been done to give correct and dependable facts. no guarantees of any sort are declared.

readers accept that the author is not involved in rendering of legal advice, professional counsel or medical advice. the material inside this book has been gathered from numerous sources.
please contact a professional before trying any tactics discussed in this book.
by reading this document, the reader accepts that under no circumstances is the author liable for any damages, direct or indirect which suffered as a consequence of the material utilized within this book including but not limited to, mistakes, omissions, or inaccuracies.

Table of content

IV. Dynamic balance exercises for seniors

A: Standing leg swings
B: Toe raises
C: Knee raises
D: Side leg raises
E: Lunges

V. Proprioceptive exercises for seniors

A: Foam pad exercises
B: Balance board exercises
C: BOSU ball exercises
E: Wobble board exercises

VI. Tai chi and yoga for seniors

A: Overview of tai chi and yoga
B: Benefits of tai chi and yoga for balance
C: Examples of tai chi and yoga poses for seniors

I. Introduction

As we age, maintaining balance becomes increasingly important for overall health and wellbeing. Seniors may experience a decline in balance due to a variety of factors such as reduced muscle strength, vision changes, and medication side effects. However, incorporating balance exercises into a fitness routine can help improve balance and prevent falls, which can be particularly dangerous for seniors. In this guide, we will explore various types of balance exercises that are safe and effective for seniors, including static and dynamic exercises, proprioceptive exercises, and tai chi and yoga. We will also provide safety tips to help prevent falls and promote a healthy and active lifestyle for seniors.

A: Why balance is important for seniors

As we age, our bodies undergo many changes, including changes to our balance. For seniors, maintaining good balance is crucial for a number of reasons, including preventing falls and maintaining independence.

One of the biggest concerns for seniors is falls. Falls are a leading cause of injury among older adults, with one in three adults over the age of 65 experiencing a fall each year. Falls can lead to serious injuries such as broken bones and head trauma, and can even be life-threatening. For seniors, falls can also lead to a loss of independence, as they may be unable to perform daily activities on their own or may require long-term care.

Maintaining good balance can help prevent falls and keep seniors independent. By incorporating balance exercises into a fitness routine, seniors can improve their overall balance and reduce their risk of falling. Balance exercises can also help improve strength, flexibility, and coordination, which can further reduce the risk of falls.

In addition to preventing falls, maintaining good balance can also improve overall health and wellbeing for seniors. Good balance can help improve posture, reduce back pain, and increase mobility. It can also help seniors maintain their ability to perform daily activities such as walking, climbing stairs, and getting in and out of chairs or beds.

There are many factors that can affect balance in seniors. These may include muscle weakness, vision changes, medication side effects, and changes in the inner ear that affect balance. By incorporating balance exercises into their fitness routine, seniors can improve their balance and reduce their risk of falls, regardless of the underlying cause of their balance issues.

Incorporating balance exercises into a fitness routine does not have to be difficult or time-consuming. There are many simple exercises that can be done at home or in a fitness class, such as standing on one leg or walking heel-to-toe. Seniors may also benefit from more advanced exercises such as yoga or tai chi, which can help improve balance and promote relaxation.

It is important for seniors to consult with their healthcare provider before starting any new exercise routine, especially if they have underlying health conditions or are taking medications that may affect their balance. In some cases, a physical therapist may be able to provide guidance on the best exercises for a senior's individual needs.

Maintaining good balance is important for seniors to prevent falls and maintain independence. By incorporating balance exercises into a fitness routine, seniors can improve their overall balance and reduce their risk of falling. This can help improve overall health and wellbeing, as well as prevent serious injuries that can lead to a loss of independence. With the right guidance and exercise plan, seniors can maintain good balance and continue to enjoy an active and healthy lifestyle.

B: How balance exercises can improve overall health

Balance exercises are not just important for preventing falls in seniors, they can also have a positive impact on overall health and wellbeing. By improving balance, seniors can improve their posture, flexibility, and strength, which can lead to better overall health.

One way that balance exercises can improve overall health is by reducing the risk of chronic diseases. According to the Centers for Disease Control and Prevention (CDC), falls are a leading cause of injury among older adults and can lead to a variety of chronic conditions, including osteoporosis, arthritis, and chronic pain. By improving balance and reducing the risk of falls, seniors may be able to prevent or manage these conditions.

Balance exercises can also improve cardiovascular health. Activities that require balance, such as yoga or tai chi, can increase heart rate and improve blood flow. This can help reduce the risk of heart disease and stroke, which are common health concerns among older adults.

In addition to physical health benefits, balance exercises can also improve mental health. Activities such as yoga or tai chi are known to promote relaxation and reduce stress. This can help improve mental wellbeing and reduce the risk of depression and anxiety.

Balance exercises can also improve cognitive function. According to a study published in the Journal of Aging and Physical Activity, balance training can improve cognitive function in older adults. This may be because balance exercises require a certain level of concentration and focus, which can help improve cognitive skills such as attention and memory.

Finally, balance exercises can improve quality of life for seniors. By reducing the risk of falls and improving overall health, seniors may be able to maintain their independence and continue to enjoy activities they love. This can lead to a better quality of life and a more positive outlook on aging.

There are many different types of balance exercises that can improve overall health in seniors. These may include static exercises, such as standing on one leg, or dynamic exercises, such as leg swings or lunges. Proprioceptive exercises, which involve using unstable surfaces such as a foam pad or balance board, can also be effective. Seniors may also benefit from activities such as yoga or tai chi, which can provide both physical and mental health benefits.

It is important for seniors to consult with their healthcare provider before starting any new exercise routine, especially if they have underlying health conditions or are taking medications that may affect their balance. A physical therapist may also be able to provide guidance on the best exercises for a senior's individual needs.

Balance exercises can have a positive impact on overall health and wellbeing in seniors. By reducing the risk of falls and improving cardiovascular health, cognitive function, and mental wellbeing, seniors may be able to maintain their independence and enjoy a better quality of life. With the right guidance and exercise plan, seniors can improve their balance and continue to enjoy an active and healthy lifestyle.

II. Types of balance exercises for seniors

A: Static balance exercises

Static balance exercises are a type of exercise that can improve balance and stability in seniors. These exercises involve maintaining a stationary position, such as standing on one leg or holding a yoga pose, for a period of time. Static balance exercises can help seniors improve their core strength, posture, and overall balance, which can reduce the risk of falls and improve overall quality of life.

One of the most basic static balance exercises for seniors is standing on one leg. To perform this exercise, seniors should stand near a wall or sturdy chair for support and lift one leg off the ground. They should try to maintain their balance for 10-15 seconds before switching legs. Seniors can gradually increase the amount of time they spend standing on one leg as they build strength and balance.

Another simple static balance exercise is heel-to-toe walking. Seniors should stand with their feet touching and one foot in front of the other, as if they are walking on a tightrope. They should then take small steps forward, placing the heel of the front foot against the toes of the back foot with each step. This exercise can help improve balance and coordination.

Seniors can also perform static balance exercises using a balance board or stability ball. These exercises involve standing on an unstable surface, which can challenge balance and improve core strength. To perform a balance board exercise, seniors should stand on the board with their feet shoulder-width apart and try to maintain their balance for 10-15 seconds. They can then try to shift their weight from side to side or front to back to further challenge their balance.

Yoga poses are also a great way for seniors to improve static balance. The tree pose, for example, involves standing on one leg and placing the sole of the other foot against the inner thigh of the standing leg. Seniors can then raise their arms overhead and hold the pose for several breaths before switching sides. Other yoga poses that can improve balance include the warrior III pose and the eagle pose.

It is important for seniors to perform static balance exercises regularly in order to see improvement. These exercises should be performed at least two to three times per week, with a goal of working up to 30 minutes of exercise per session. Seniors should also be sure to warm up before performing static balance exercises and cool down afterward to prevent injury.

Overall, static balance exercises are a safe and effective way for seniors to improve balance and stability. These exercises can be performed at home with little or no equipment, making them an accessible option for many seniors. By incorporating static balance exercises into their exercise routine, seniors can improve their overall quality of life and reduce the risk of falls and injuries.

B: Dynamic balance exercises

Dynamic balance exercises are a type of exercise that can improve balance and stability in seniors by incorporating movement. These exercises involve moving while maintaining balance, such as walking heel-to-toe or stepping over obstacles. Dynamic balance exercises can help seniors improve their coordination, reaction time, and overall balance, which can reduce the risk of falls and improve overall quality of life.

One of the most basic dynamic balance exercises for seniors is the single-leg reach. To perform this exercise, seniors should stand with their feet shoulder-width apart and lift one leg off the ground. They should then reach forward with the opposite hand and touch the toes of the lifted leg before returning to the starting position. Seniors can then repeat the exercise on the other side. This exercise can be modified to increase difficulty by using a resistance band or adding a hop at the end of the reach.

Another simple dynamic balance exercise is walking sideways. Seniors should stand with their feet shoulder-width apart and take several steps to the side, keeping their toes pointed forward. They should then return to the starting position and repeat the exercise in the other direction. This exercise can help improve coordination and balance while also targeting the muscles in the legs and hips.

Seniors can also perform dynamic balance exercises using a balance board or stability ball. These exercises involve standing on an unstable surface while performing movements such as squats or lunges. To perform a balance board exercise, seniors should stand on the board with their feet shoulder-width apart and perform a squat or lunge while maintaining their balance. They can then try to shift their weight from side to side or front to back to further challenge their balance.

Dancing is also a fun and effective way for seniors to improve dynamic balance. Seniors can participate in dance classes that focus on balance and coordination, such as ballroom dancing or salsa dancing. These classes can help seniors improve their balance while also providing a social outlet and improving their mood.

It is important for seniors to perform dynamic balance exercises regularly in order to see improvement. These exercises should be performed at least two to three times per week, with a goal of working up to 30 minutes of exercise per session. Seniors should also be sure to warm up before performing dynamic balance exercises and cool down afterward to prevent injury.

Overall, dynamic balance exercises are a safe and effective way for seniors to improve balance and stability. These exercises can be performed at home with little or no equipment, making them an accessible option for many seniors. By incorporating dynamic balance exercises into their exercise routine, seniors can improve their overall quality of life and reduce the risk of falls and injuries.

C: Proprioceptive exercises

Proprioceptive exercises are a type of balance exercise that focus on improving a senior's ability to sense the position and movement of their body. These exercises can help seniors improve their balance and coordination, reduce the risk of falls, and improve overall mobility.

One common proprioceptive exercise for seniors is standing on one leg with their eyes closed. Seniors should stand with their feet hip-width apart and lift one foot off the ground. They should then close their eyes and hold the position for as long as they can before switching to the other leg. This exercise helps seniors improve their ability to sense the position of their body in space, which can improve balance and coordination.

Another proprioceptive exercise is the balance beam walk. Seniors can use a balance beam, a piece of wood, or a long strip of tape on the floor to create a narrow path. They should then walk along the path, placing one foot directly in front of the other. This exercise helps seniors improve their balance and coordination by challenging their ability to maintain their center of gravity over a narrow surface.

Seniors can also perform proprioceptive exercises using a stability ball. They can sit on the ball and perform exercises such as arm circles or leg lifts while maintaining their balance on the ball. This exercise challenges the seniors' ability to sense the position of their body in space and improve overall balance.

Another proprioceptive exercise is the heel-to-toe walk. Seniors should walk heel-to-toe in a straight line, keeping their toes pointed forward and their heel touching the toes of the other foot. This exercise improves seniors' balance and coordination by challenging their ability to maintain their center of gravity over a narrow surface.

Seniors can also perform proprioceptive exercises while standing on a soft surface such as a foam pad. They should stand with their feet hip-width apart and lift one foot off the ground. They should then place their foot on the foam pad and hold the position for as long as they can before switching to the other leg. This exercise challenges the seniors' ability to sense the position of their body in space on an unstable surface.

It is important for seniors to perform proprioceptive exercises regularly in order to see improvement. These exercises should be performed at least two to three times per week, with a goal of working up to 30 minutes of exercise per session. Seniors should also be sure to warm up before performing proprioceptive exercises and cool down afterward to prevent injury.

Proprioceptive exercises are a safe and effective way for seniors to improve their balance and coordination. These exercises can be performed at home with little or no equipment, making them an accessible option for many seniors. By incorporating proprioceptive exercises into their exercise routine, seniors can improve their overall quality of life and reduce the risk of falls and injuries.

D: Tai chi and yoga

Tai chi and yoga are two forms of exercise that can help seniors improve their balance, strength, and flexibility. Both of these exercises are low-impact and can be adapted to suit seniors of all fitness levels and abilities.

Tai chi is a Chinese martial art that is often practiced for its health benefits. Tai chi involves slow, deliberate movements that flow from one pose to the next. These movements are designed to improve balance, coordination, and flexibility. Tai chi also incorporates deep breathing exercises, which can help seniors reduce stress and improve relaxation.

Research has shown that tai chi can help seniors improve their balance and reduce the risk of falls. One study found that seniors who practiced tai chi regularly had a 47% reduction in falls compared to those who did not practice tai chi. Tai chi can also help seniors improve their overall physical function, such as the ability to perform activities of daily living.

Yoga is another form of exercise that can be beneficial for seniors. Yoga involves a series of poses, breathing exercises, and meditation. Yoga can help seniors improve their flexibility, balance, and strength. Yoga also has mental health benefits, such as reducing stress and anxiety.

Research has shown that yoga can be effective for improving balance in seniors.

One study found that seniors who practiced yoga had better balance and lower rates of falls compared to those who did not practice yoga. Yoga can also improve flexibility and joint mobility, which can help seniors maintain their independence and improve their quality of life.

Seniors who are interested in practicing tai chi or yoga should start with a beginner's class. These classes are designed to introduce seniors to the basic poses and movements of each exercise. Seniors should also consult with their doctor before starting any new exercise program to ensure that it is safe for them.

It is important for seniors to practice tai chi or yoga regularly in order to see improvement. Ideally, seniors should practice these exercises at least two to three times per week for 30 to 60 minutes per session. Seniors should also be sure to warm up before starting their practice and cool down afterward to prevent injury.

Tai chi and yoga are two forms of exercise that can be beneficial for seniors. These exercises can help seniors improve their balance, flexibility, and strength, as well as reduce the risk of falls. Seniors who are interested in practicing tai chi or yoga should start with a beginner's class and consult with their doctor before starting any new exercise program. With regular practice, seniors can improve their overall physical function and quality of life.

III. Static balance exercises for seniors

A: One-legged stand

The one-legged stand is a simple but effective balance exercise that can be done by seniors to improve their balance and stability. This exercise can be done anywhere and doesn't require any equipment, making it a convenient option for seniors who want to incorporate balance exercises into their daily routine.

To perform the one-legged stand, seniors should stand on one leg with their arms at their sides. They should hold this position for as long as possible, aiming for at least 30 seconds before switching to the other leg. As seniors become more comfortable with this exercise, they can increase the duration of each hold.

The one-legged stand can be challenging at first, but it is an effective exercise for improving balance and stability. This exercise can help seniors strengthen the muscles in their feet, ankles, and legs, which are important for maintaining balance and preventing falls.

In addition to strengthening the muscles in the lower body, the one-legged stand also helps seniors improve their proprioception, which is the ability to sense the position and movement of their body in space. Proprioception is an important factor in balance and stability, and can deteriorate with age or injury. By practicing the one-legged stand, seniors can improve their proprioception and reduce the risk of falls.

It's important for seniors to start slowly with the one-legged stand and gradually increase the duration of each hold. Seniors can also vary the difficulty of this exercise by standing on a soft surface, such as a foam pad, or by holding onto a stable surface, such as a chair or countertop. Seniors should also ensure that they have a clear space around them and that they are wearing appropriate footwear with good traction.

The one-legged stand is a simple but effective balance exercise that can be done by seniors to improve their balance and stability. This exercise can be incorporated into a daily routine and doesn't require any equipment, making it a convenient option for seniors who want to improve their balance. By practicing the one-legged stand regularly, seniors can strengthen the muscles in their lower body, improve their proprioception, and reduce the risk of falls.

B: Heel-to-toe stand

The heel-to-toe stand is a balance exercise that is particularly helpful for improving gait and reducing the risk of falls in seniors.

This exercise challenges the senior's balance, coordination, and proprioception, which can help seniors improve their overall mobility and confidence.

To perform the heel-to-toe stand, seniors should stand with their feet together and then place one foot directly in front of the other so that the heel of the front foot touches the toes of the back foot. Seniors should then take a step forward with the back foot and place it directly in front of the front foot, continuing this heel-to-toe movement as they walk a straight line.

The heel-to-toe stand can be made more challenging by incorporating turns or walking backward. This exercise can also be performed with the senior's eyes closed, which can further challenge their balance and proprioception.

The heel-to-toe stand is particularly helpful for improving gait and reducing the risk of falls in seniors. By practicing this exercise regularly, seniors can improve their balance and coordination, which can lead to more confident and stable movement. This can help seniors maintain their independence and quality of life as they age.

It's important for seniors to start slowly with the heel-to-toe stand and gradually increase the difficulty of the exercise. Seniors should also ensure that they have a clear space around them and that they are wearing appropriate footwear with good traction. A stable surface, such as a countertop or chair, can also be used for support as needed.

In addition to improving balance and coordination, the heel-to-toe stand can also provide a low-impact workout for the legs and core. Seniors can also incorporate this exercise into their daily routine, such as walking down a hallway or around the house.

Overall, the heel-to-toe stand is an effective and low-impact balance exercise that can be done by seniors to improve their gait and reduce the risk of falls. This exercise can be adapted to the senior's level of fitness and mobility, making it a convenient and versatile option for seniors who want to incorporate balance exercises into their daily routine.

C: Tightrope walk

The tightrope walk is a challenging balance exercise that can help seniors improve their balance, coordination, and proprioception. This exercise involves walking along a line that is taped or painted on the ground, mimicking the movement of walking along a tightrope.

To perform the tightrope walk, seniors should first find a clear space with a straight line on the ground. They should then stand with their feet together and raise their arms out to the sides for balance. Seniors should then begin to take steps along the line, placing one foot directly in front of the other and maintaining their balance as they move forward.

The tightrope walk can be made more challenging by incorporating turns, walking backward, or even adding obstacles such as cones or small objects to step over. Seniors can also try performing this exercise with their eyes closed to further challenge their balance and proprioception.

The tightrope walk is a great exercise for seniors because it not only helps to improve balance and coordination, but it also strengthens the muscles in the legs and core. This can lead to better stability and mobility, which can reduce the risk of falls and improve overall quality of life.

When performing the tightrope walk, it's important for seniors to start slowly and focus on maintaining their balance and form. They should also make sure that the surface they are walking on is stable and not slippery, and that they are wearing shoes with good traction.

Seniors can incorporate the tightrope walk into their daily routine by practicing in their home or in a safe outdoor area. They can also make it a fun activity to do with friends or family members, which can help to keep them motivated and engaged in their balance exercise routine.

The tightrope walk is a challenging and effective balance exercise that can help seniors improve their balance, coordination, and proprioception. By incorporating this exercise into their daily routine, seniors can strengthen their muscles, reduce the risk of falls, and maintain their independence and quality of life.

D: Stork stand

The stork stand is a balance exercise that can help seniors improve their stability and strengthen the muscles in their legs and core. This exercise involves standing on one leg and lifting the opposite knee up towards the chest while maintaining balance.

To perform the stork stand, seniors should first find a clear space with a sturdy chair or counter for support if needed. They should then stand with their feet together and lift one foot off the ground, bending the knee and bringing it up towards the chest. Seniors should hold this position for several seconds, maintaining their balance and keeping their core engaged.

As seniors become more comfortable with this exercise, they can try holding the position for longer periods of time or incorporating small movements, such as lifting and lowering the lifted leg or rotating the ankle. Seniors can also try performing the stork stand with their eyes closed to further challenge their balance and proprioception.

The stork stand is a great exercise for seniors because it not only helps to improve balance and stability, but it also strengthens the muscles in the legs and core. This can lead to better posture and reduced risk of falls, which can improve overall quality of life.

When performing the stork stand, seniors should start slowly and focus on maintaining their balance and form. They should also make sure that the surface they are standing on is stable and not slippery, and that they are wearing shoes with good traction.

Seniors can incorporate the stork stand into their daily routine by practicing in their home or in a safe outdoor area. They can also make it a fun activity to do with friends or family members, which can help to keep them motivated and engaged in their balance exercise routine.

The stork stand is an effective balance exercise that can help seniors improve their stability and strengthen the muscles in their legs and core. By incorporating this exercise into their daily routine, seniors can reduce the risk of falls, improve their posture, and maintain their independence and quality of life.

E: Flamingo stand

The flamingo stand is a balance exercise that can be beneficial for seniors who want to improve their stability, posture, and overall fitness. This exercise involves standing on one leg and extending the other leg backwards, resembling a flamingo standing on one leg.

To perform the flamingo stand, seniors should first find a clear space with a sturdy chair or counter for support if needed. They should then stand with their feet together and lift one foot off the ground, bending the knee and bringing it up towards the chest. Next, seniors should extend the lifted leg backwards, keeping it straight and parallel to the ground. They should hold this position for several seconds, maintaining their balance and keeping their core engaged.

As seniors become more comfortable with this exercise, they can try holding the position for longer periods of time or incorporating small movements, such as lifting and lowering the lifted leg or rotating the ankle. Seniors can also try performing the flamingo stand with their eyes closed to further challenge their balance and proprioception.

The flamingo stand is a great exercise for seniors because it not only helps to improve balance and stability, but it also strengthens the muscles in the legs, core, and back. This can lead to better posture, reduced risk of falls, and improved overall fitness.

When performing the flamingo stand, seniors should start slowly and focus on maintaining their balance and form. They should also make sure that the surface they are standing on is stable and not slippery, and that they are wearing shoes with good traction.

Seniors can incorporate the flamingo stand into their daily routine by practicing in their home or in a safe outdoor area. They can also make it a fun activity to do with friends or family members, which can help to keep them motivated and engaged in their balance exercise routine.

The flamingo stand is an effective balance exercise that can help seniors improve their stability, posture, and overall fitness. By incorporating this exercise into their daily routine, seniors can reduce the risk of falls, improve their quality of life, and maintain their independence.

IV. Dynamic balance exercises for seniors

A: Standing leg swings

Standing leg swings are a simple yet effective balance exercise that can benefit seniors who want to improve their stability and flexibility. This exercise involves swinging one leg forward and backward while standing on the other leg.

To perform standing leg swings, seniors should start by standing with their feet shoulder-width apart and their hands on their hips or holding onto a sturdy object for balance. They should then shift their weight onto one leg and swing the other leg forward and backward, keeping it straight and parallel to the ground. Seniors should aim to swing the leg as high as they comfortably can, while maintaining their balance and keeping their core engaged. They can repeat this motion for several swings before switching to the other leg.

Seniors can also perform standing leg swings with a lateral motion, swinging the leg from side to side instead of forward and backward. This can help to improve balance and stability in different directions and engage different muscle groups.

Standing leg swings are a great exercise for seniors because they help to improve balance and stability, as well as flexibility in the hips and legs. This can lead to better posture, reduced risk of falls, and improved overall fitness.

When performing standing leg swings, seniors should start slowly and focus on maintaining their balance and form. They should also make sure that the surface they are standing on is stable and not slippery, and that they are wearing shoes with good traction.

Seniors can incorporate standing leg swings into their daily routine by practicing in their home or in a safe outdoor area. They can also make it a fun activity to do with friends or family members, which can help to keep them motivated and engaged in their balance exercise routine.

Standing leg swings are an effective and simple balance exercise that can help seniors improve their stability, flexibility, and overall fitness. By incorporating this exercise into their daily routine, seniors can reduce the risk of falls, improve their quality of life, and maintain their independence.

B: Toe raises

Toe raises are a simple yet effective balance exercise that can benefit seniors who want to improve their strength and stability in the feet, ankles, and lower legs. This exercise involves lifting the heels off the ground while standing on the balls of the feet.

To perform toe raises, seniors should start by standing with their feet shoulder-width apart and their hands on their hips or holding onto a sturdy object for balance. They should then shift their weight onto the balls of their feet, lifting their heels off the ground as high as they comfortably can. Seniors should aim to keep their toes pointed forward and their ankles stable throughout the exercise. They can hold this position for a few seconds before lowering their heels back down to the ground.

Seniors can repeat toe raises for several repetitions, gradually increasing the number of repetitions as their strength and balance improve.

Toe raises are a great exercise for seniors because they help to improve the strength and stability of the feet, ankles, and lower legs. This can lead to improved balance, reduced risk of falls, and improved overall fitness.

When performing toe raises, seniors should start slowly and focus on maintaining their balance and form. They should also make sure that the surface they are standing on is stable and not slippery, and that they are wearing shoes with good traction.

Seniors can incorporate toe raises into their daily routine by practicing in their home or in a safe outdoor area. They can also make it a fun activity to do with friends or family members, which can help to keep them motivated and engaged in their balance exercise routine.

Toe raises are an effective and simple balance exercise that can help seniors improve their strength, stability, and overall fitness. By incorporating this exercise into their daily routine, seniors can reduce the risk of falls, improve their quality of life, and maintain their independence.

C: Knee raises

Knee raises are a simple yet effective exercise that can help seniors improve their balance, stability, and overall fitness. This exercise involves lifting one knee up towards the chest while standing on one leg.

To perform knee raises, seniors should start by standing with their feet shoulder-width apart and their hands on their hips or holding onto a sturdy object for balance. They should then shift their weight onto one leg and lift the opposite knee up towards the chest. Seniors should aim to keep their toes pointed forward and their hips level throughout the exercise. They can hold this position for a few seconds before lowering their leg back down to the ground.

Seniors can repeat knee raises for several repetitions on each leg, gradually increasing the number of repetitions as their strength and balance improve.

Knee raises are a great exercise for seniors because they help to improve the strength and stability of the hips, thighs, and core muscles. This can lead to improved balance, reduced risk of falls, and improved overall fitness.

When performing knee raises, seniors should start slowly and focus on maintaining their balance and form. They should also make sure that the surface they are standing on is stable and not slippery, and that they are wearing shoes with good traction.

Seniors can incorporate knee raises into their daily routine by practicing in their home or in a safe outdoor area. They can also make it a fun activity to do with friends or family members, which can help to keep them motivated and engaged in their balance exercise routine.

Overall, knee raises are an effective and simple balance exercise that can help seniors improve their strength, stability, and overall fitness. By incorporating this exercise into their daily routine, seniors can reduce the risk of falls, improve their quality of life, and maintain their independence.

D: Side leg raises

Side leg raises are an excellent exercise that can help seniors improve their balance, stability, and overall fitness. This exercise targets the muscles of the hips and thighs, which are crucial for maintaining balance and preventing falls.

To perform side leg raises, seniors should start by standing with their feet shoulder-width apart and their hands on their hips or holding onto a sturdy object for balance. They should then shift their weight onto one leg and lift the opposite leg out to the side, keeping their toes pointed forward and their hips level. Seniors should aim to lift their leg as high as they comfortably can while maintaining good form. They can hold this position for a few seconds before lowering their leg back down to the ground.

Seniors can repeat side leg raises for several repetitions on each leg, gradually increasing the number of repetitions as their strength and balance improve.

Side leg raises are a great exercise for seniors because they help to improve the strength and stability of the hips and thighs, which are crucial for maintaining balance and preventing falls. This exercise also helps to improve flexibility in the hip muscles, which can reduce the risk of hip injuries.

When performing side leg raises, seniors should start slowly and focus on maintaining good form and balance. They should also make sure that the surface they are standing on is stable and not slippery, and that they are wearing shoes with good traction.

Seniors can incorporate side leg raises into their daily routine by practicing in their home or in a safe outdoor area. They can also make it a fun activity to do with friends or family members, which can help to keep them motivated and engaged in their balance exercise routine.

Side leg raises are an effective and simple balance exercise that can help seniors improve their strength, stability, and overall fitness. By incorporating this exercise into their daily routine, seniors can reduce the risk of falls, improve their quality of life, and maintain their independence.

E: Lunges

Lunges are an excellent exercise for seniors looking to improve their balance, strength, and overall fitness. This exercise targets the muscles of the lower body, including the quads, hamstrings, and glutes, which are essential for maintaining stability and preventing falls.

To perform lunges, seniors should start by standing with their feet hip-width apart and their hands on their hips or holding onto a sturdy object for balance. They should then step forward with one leg, bending their knee to lower their body down towards the ground. The front knee should be directly over the ankle, and the back knee should lower towards the ground without touching it. Seniors should aim to keep their back straight and their core engaged throughout the movement. They can then push off the front foot and return to a standing position before repeating the lunge with the opposite leg.

Seniors can repeat lunges for several repetitions on each leg, gradually increasing the number of repetitions as their strength and balance improve.

Lunges are a great exercise for seniors because they help to improve the strength and stability of the lower body, which is crucial for maintaining balance and preventing falls. This exercise also helps to improve flexibility in the hips and knees, which can reduce the risk of injuries.

When performing lunges, seniors should start slowly and focus on maintaining good form and balance. They should also make sure that the surface they are standing on is stable and not slippery, and that they are wearing shoes with good traction.

Seniors can incorporate lunges into their daily routine by practicing in their home or in a safe outdoor area. They can also make it a fun activity to do with friends or family members, which can help to keep them motivated and engaged in their balance exercise routine.

Lunges are an effective and challenging balance exercise that can help seniors improve their strength, stability, and overall fitness. By incorporating this exercise into their daily routine, seniors can reduce the risk of falls, improve their quality of life, and maintain their independence.

V. Proprioceptive exercises for seniors

A: Foam pad exercises

Foam pad exercises are an excellent way for seniors to improve their balance and stability. These exercises involve performing various movements on a foam pad, which provides an unstable surface that challenges the body's balance and coordination.

Foam pads come in various shapes and sizes, but most are rectangular or square and made of a soft, spongy material. The pads are designed to be unstable, making it challenging for seniors to maintain their balance and control while performing different movements.

Foam pad exercises can be performed in a variety of ways, depending on the senior's fitness level and mobility. Some popular foam pad exercises for seniors include:

Balance beam: seniors can practice walking forwards, backwards, and sideways along the foam pad as if they were walking along a balance beam. This exercise helps to improve overall balance, coordination, and lower body strength.

Single-leg stance: seniors can stand on one foot on the foam pad for as long as possible before switching to the other foot. This exercise helps to improve balance, stability, and lower body strength.

Squats: seniors can perform squats on the foam pad by standing on the pad with their feet hip-width apart and squatting down as low as they can before standing up again. This exercise helps to improve lower body strength and balance.

Tandem stance: seniors can stand with one foot in front of the other on the foam pad, with the heel of the back foot touching the toes of the front foot. This exercise helps to improve overall balance and stability.

Foam pad exercises are beneficial for seniors for several reasons. First, they help to improve balance and stability, which can reduce the risk of falls and injuries. These exercises also challenge the body's proprioception, or sense of where the body is in space, which can help seniors maintain their independence and mobility.

Additionally, foam pad exercises can be adapted to suit a range of fitness levels and abilities, making them suitable for seniors with varying levels of mobility and balance. They can also be performed at home with minimal equipment, making them a convenient and accessible exercise option for seniors.

However, it's important for seniors to start slowly with foam pad exercises and to gradually increase the difficulty of the exercises as their balance and coordination improve. Seniors should also ensure they have adequate support and stability when performing foam pad exercises, such as holding onto a sturdy object or having a caregiver nearby for assistance.

Foam pad exercises are a fun and effective way for seniors to improve their balance, stability, and overall fitness. By incorporating these exercises into their daily routine, seniors can reduce their risk of falls, improve their quality of life, and maintain their independence.

B: Balance board exercises

Balance board exercises are an effective way for seniors to improve their balance and stability. These exercises involve standing on a board that is designed to be unstable, which forces the user to engage their core muscles and make constant adjustments to maintain balance.

There are several types of balance boards available, including wobble boards, rocker boards, and balance disks. Each type of board provides a different level of challenge and can be used for different exercises.

One of the most basic balance board exercises is simply standing on the board with both feet and trying to maintain balance. As the user becomes more comfortable, they can progress to more challenging exercises such as:

Single-leg balance: Stand on one leg on the balance board, holding onto a stable object if necessary. Once this becomes easy, try performing the exercise with your eyes closed.

Side-to-side balance: Stand on the board with feet hip-width apart and shift your weight from side to side, using your core muscles to maintain balance.

Front-to-back balance: Stand on the board with feet hip-width apart and shift your weight forward and backward, using your core muscles to maintain balance.

Squats: Stand on the board with feet shoulder-width apart and slowly lower into a squat position, using your core muscles to maintain balance.

Lunges: Stand on the board with one foot on the center of the board and the other foot on the ground. Slowly lower into a lunge position, using your core muscles to maintain balance.

Balance board exercises can be performed at home or in a gym setting with the guidance of a trainer. They are a great way for seniors to improve their balance, stability, and overall fitness.

C: BOSU ball exercises

The BOSU ball is a versatile piece of equipment that can be used to perform a wide range of balance exercises for seniors. The BOSU ball is essentially half of a stability ball with a flat platform on one side and a dome-shaped surface on the other. This design allows for a variety of exercises that target different muscle groups and improve overall balance and stability.

Here are some BOSU ball exercises that seniors can try:

Balance on the dome: Start by standing on the dome side of the BOSU ball with feet hip-width apart. Try to maintain balance for 30-60 seconds. As this exercise becomes easier, progress to single-leg balance or closing your eyes while balancing.

Squats: Stand on the flat side of the BOSU ball with feet shoulder-width apart. Slowly lower into a squat position, using your core muscles to maintain balance. As this exercise becomes easier, add weight by holding dumbbells or a medicine ball.

Lunges: Stand on the flat side of the BOSU ball with one foot on the center of the ball and the other foot on the ground. Slowly lower into a lunge position, using your core muscles to maintain balance. Repeat with the other leg.

Push-ups: Place the BOSU ball on the ground with the dome side up. Place your hands on the edges of the dome and lower your body into a push-up position, keeping your core engaged.

Plank: Place the BOSU ball on the ground with the dome side down. Place your forearms on the center of the dome and extend your legs behind you, keeping your body in a straight line and your core engaged.

BOSU ball exercises can be modified to suit any fitness level and can be performed in a gym or at home. They are a great way for seniors to improve their balance, stability, and overall fitness. Regular practice of these exercises can help seniors maintain their independence, prevent falls, and improve their quality of life.

D: Wobble board exercises

Wobble boards are a popular piece of equipment used for balance training, particularly in rehabilitation settings. A wobble board is essentially a circular board with a hemisphere on the bottom, which creates an unstable surface that challenges the user's balance.

Wobble board exercises are an effective way to improve balance, stability, and core strength. They can be done in a variety of ways to target different muscle groups and challenge different aspects of balance.

One of the most basic wobble board exercises is simply standing on the board with both feet and trying to maintain balance. Once this becomes easy, the user can progress to standing on one foot, or closing their eyes while standing on the board. This exercise can be made more challenging by adding arm movements or performing squats or lunges while standing on the board.

Another common wobble board exercise is the "figure eight." This involves standing on the board and moving it in a figure-eight pattern with the feet, while maintaining balance. This exercise targets the muscles of the lower body, as well as the core, and can help to improve balance and coordination.

A similar exercise is the "clock face." This involves standing on the board and moving the feet in a circular pattern around the edge of the board, as if tracing the numbers of a clock face. This exercise targets the muscles of the lower legs and feet, and can help to improve balance and stability.

For a more challenging exercise, the user can try performing push-ups on the wobble board. This exercise not only challenges the muscles of the upper body, but also requires significant core strength and balance to perform correctly.

Wobble board exercises can also be combined with other exercises, such as lunges or squats, to create a more challenging and dynamic workout. For example, performing a lunge while holding a weight in one hand and standing on the wobble board with the opposite foot requires significant core strength and balance, as well as strength in the legs and upper body.

Wobble board exercises are an effective way to improve balance, stability, and core strength. They can be done in a variety of ways to target different muscle groups and challenge different aspects of balance. When used regularly as part of a balanced exercise program, wobble board exercises can help seniors to maintain their independence and reduce the risk of falls.

VI. Tai chi and yoga for seniors

A: Overview of tai chi and yoga

Tai Chi and yoga are two popular exercise programs that have been shown to provide numerous benefits for seniors. Both of these practices incorporate slow, controlled movements that promote balance, flexibility, and strength, making them ideal for seniors looking to improve their overall health and well-being.

Tai Chi is a Chinese martial art that has been practiced for centuries. It involves a series of flowing movements that are performed in a slow, deliberate manner. Tai Chi is often referred to as "moving meditation" because it requires focus and concentration, which can have a calming effect on the mind and body. Tai Chi has been shown to improve balance, reduce the risk of falls, and increase flexibility and strength. It has also been linked to a reduction in symptoms of depression and anxiety, as well as improvements in sleep quality.

Yoga is a practice that originated in ancient India and has become popular worldwide. It involves a series of postures, or asanas, that are designed to promote strength, flexibility, and balance. Yoga also emphasizes the importance of breathing techniques and relaxation, which can help reduce stress and promote overall well-being. Like Tai Chi, yoga has been shown to improve balance and reduce the risk of falls in seniors. It has also been linked to improvements in flexibility, strength, and cardiovascular health.

Both Tai Chi and yoga can be modified to accommodate seniors of all fitness levels and abilities. They can be practiced in a group setting or at home with the use of instructional videos or classes. Some seniors may prefer one practice over the other, but both can be effective in improving balance and overall health.

Tai Chi and yoga are two popular exercise programs that provide numerous benefits for seniors. They promote balance, flexibility, and strength, and can be modified to accommodate seniors of all fitness levels and abilities. Practicing Tai Chi or yoga can have a positive impact on both physical and mental health, making them excellent options for seniors looking to improve their overall well-being.

B: Benefits of tai chi and yoga for balance

Tai chi and yoga are both ancient practices that have become increasingly popular for their numerous health benefits, including improving balance in seniors. These practices are low-impact and focus on the mind-body connection, making them accessible to people of all ages and fitness levels.

Tai chi is a Chinese martial art that consists of a series of slow, flowing movements that emphasize balance, coordination, and mindfulness. It has been shown to improve balance, reduce the risk of falls, and improve overall physical function in seniors. In fact, a systematic review of 10 randomized controlled trials found that tai chi reduced the risk of falls by 43% in older adults. Tai chi also helps to improve muscle strength, flexibility, and range of motion, all of which contribute to better balance.

Yoga is a practice that originated in ancient India and involves a series of poses and breathing exercises that promote relaxation, flexibility, and balance. Yoga has been shown to improve balance in seniors by increasing strength, flexibility, and body awareness. Additionally, yoga can help to reduce stress and anxiety, which can contribute to better balance by improving focus and concentration.

One of the main benefits of tai chi and yoga for balance is that they both focus on improving proprioception, or the body's ability to sense its position in space. This is particularly important for seniors, as proprioception naturally declines with age, leading to increased falls risk. Both practices require participants to maintain balance while shifting their weight, which helps to improve proprioception and reduce the risk of falls.

Another benefit of tai chi and yoga for balance is that they can be modified to meet the needs and abilities of each individual. Instructors can provide variations of poses or movements, or use props such as chairs or blocks to make the practice more accessible for those with limited mobility or balance issues.

Overall, tai chi and yoga are both excellent practices for improving balance in seniors.

They are low-impact, accessible, and provide numerous physical and mental health benefits in addition to improving balance. Seniors who are interested in incorporating these practices into their exercise routine should speak with their healthcare provider to ensure that it is safe for them to do so, and work with a qualified instructor to ensure that they are using proper form and technique.

C: Examples of tai chi and yoga poses for seniors

Tai chi and yoga are both excellent forms of exercise for seniors to improve balance and overall well-being. They both focus on slow, deliberate movements and breathing techniques that can help improve flexibility, strength, and balance.

Here are some examples of tai chi and yoga poses that are particularly beneficial for seniors:

Tai Chi: "Cloud Hands" - This involves shifting your weight from one foot to the other while making slow, circular movements with your arms.

Yoga: "Mountain Pose" - Stand tall with your feet hip-width apart, arms at your sides, and shoulders relaxed. Focus on your breathing as you lift your arms overhead and hold the pose.

Tai Chi: "Single Whip" - This involves stepping forward with one foot while simultaneously raising one arm and lowering the other.

Yoga: "Warrior II" - Stand with your feet wide apart, arms outstretched, and bend your front knee while keeping your back leg straight. This pose can help improve balance and strengthen the legs.

Tai Chi: "Needle at Sea Bottom" - This involves bending forward and reaching down with one hand while raising the other behind you.

Yoga: "Tree Pose" - Stand with one foot pressed against the inside of your opposite leg, and your hands in a prayer position at your chest. This pose can help improve balance and strengthen the leg muscles.

Tai Chi: "Snake Creeps Down" - This involves bending forward while keeping your back straight and reaching down with both hands.

Yoga: "Chair Pose" - Stand with your feet hip-width apart and raise your arms overhead while bending your knees as if you are sitting in a chair. This pose can help improve balance and strengthen the leg muscles.

Tai Chi: "Golden Rooster Stands on One Leg" - This involves balancing on one foot while lifting the other leg and raising one arm.

Yoga: "Downward Dog" - Start on all fours with your hands and knees on the ground, and then lift your hips up while straightening your arms and legs. This pose can help improve balance and flexibility.

Both tai chi and yoga offer many benefits for seniors, including improved balance, strength, flexibility, and overall well-being. These exercises can be modified to meet the needs of seniors with varying levels of mobility and can be practiced in group settings or at home.

VII. Safety tips for balance exercises for seniors

A: How to prevent falls

Falls are a major concern for seniors, and preventing them is crucial to maintaining good health and independence. There are several steps seniors can take to help reduce their risk of falling:

Exercise regularly: Regular exercise, including balance and strength training, can help improve balance, coordination, and muscle strength, reducing the risk of falls.

Wear proper footwear: Shoes should fit well, have good support and a non-slip sole. Avoid high heels or shoes with slippery soles.

Keep your home safe: Remove tripping hazards such as loose rugs, clutter, and electrical cords. Install grab bars in the bathroom and handrails on stairways.

Improve lighting: Make sure there is adequate lighting throughout the home, especially in stairways, hallways, and entrances. Use night lights in bedrooms and bathrooms.

Be aware of medications: Some medications can cause dizziness, lightheadedness or sleepiness, which can increase the risk of falling. Talk to your doctor or pharmacist about the side effects of your medications.

Have your vision checked: Poor vision can increase the risk of falls. Have your eyes checked regularly and wear glasses or contact lenses as prescribed.

Be cautious: Take your time when getting up from a chair or bed, and when walking. Use handrails when going up and down stairs, and take small steps when turning.

Stay hydrated: Dehydration can cause dizziness and lightheadedness, increasing the risk of falls. Drink plenty of water throughout the day.

Get enough sleep: Lack of sleep can affect balance and coordination, increasing the risk of falls. Aim for 7-8 hours of sleep each night.

Stay active and engaged: Participating in social activities, hobbies, and other interests can help improve physical and mental health, reducing the risk of falls.

By taking these steps, seniors can reduce their risk of falling and maintain their independence and quality of life. It's important to talk to a healthcare provider about any concerns regarding falls or balance, as they can provide personalized recommendations and referrals to specialists as needed.

B: When to consult a doctor or physical therapist

Balance exercises can be incredibly beneficial for seniors, but it is important to know when to seek professional help. If you are experiencing frequent falls or have a medical condition that affects your balance, it is important to consult with a doctor or physical therapist before beginning any new exercise program.

A physical therapist can evaluate your current balance and mobility and create an individualized exercise plan tailored to your specific needs. They can also teach you proper techniques for performing balance exercises and monitor your progress over time.

Additionally, if you experience dizziness or lightheadedness during or after performing balance exercises, it is important to consult with a healthcare professional. These symptoms could be a sign of an underlying medical condition that needs to be addressed.

It is also important to note that certain medications can affect balance and increase the risk of falls. If you are taking any medications, be sure to discuss their potential side effects with your doctor or pharmacist.

Overall, if you have any concerns about your balance or mobility, it is best to consult with a healthcare professional to ensure your safety and well-being.

VIII. Conclusion

A: The importance of incorporating balance exercises into a senior's fitness routine.

Incorporating balance exercises into a senior's fitness routine is crucial for maintaining their overall health and well-being. As we age, our bodies undergo various changes that affect our balance, coordination, and stability. These changes can increase the risk of falls and injuries, leading to a decline in physical activity and a decreased quality of life.

Balance exercises help improve proprioception, which is the body's ability to sense and respond to changes in its position and movement. By doing so, these exercises help seniors maintain their balance and stability, reduce the risk of falls, and improve their confidence in performing daily activities.

In addition, incorporating balance exercises into a senior's fitness routine can have other health benefits, such as improved posture, increased flexibility, and strengthened muscles. These exercises can also improve cardiovascular health and reduce the risk of chronic conditions such as diabetes, hypertension, and obesity.

The key to reaping the benefits of balance exercises is to incorporate them into a regular fitness routine. Seniors should aim to perform these exercises at least two to three times a week, with a focus on gradually increasing the difficulty and intensity over time. It's important to note that balance exercises should be performed in a safe and controlled environment, such as a fitness center or under the guidance of a trained professional.

There are many different types of balance exercises that seniors can incorporate into their fitness routine, including static and dynamic exercises, as well as exercises using various equipment such as foam pads, balance boards, and BOSU balls. Tai chi and yoga are also great options for improving balance and stability, as they incorporate movements that require a strong focus on balance and coordination.

Overall, incorporating balance exercises into a senior's fitness routine is a crucial step in maintaining their overall health and well-being. These exercises can help improve balance, stability, posture, and flexibility, as well as reduce the risk of falls and injuries. Seniors should consult with their healthcare provider or a trained fitness professional to determine the best exercises for their individual needs and abilities.